'BY BEING YOURSELF YOU PUT SOMETHING WONDERFUL IN THE WORLD WHICH WAS NOT THERE BEFORE'
EDWIN ELLIOT

Acknowledgements:

I would like to say a huge thank you to all those of you who critiqued, proof-read and offered great suggestions for this booklet:

Richard Pearce
Naia Headland-Vanni
Anna Goodwin
Mags O'Brien
Emma Simmonds
Andrew Sceats

'STRESS SHOULD BE A POWERFUL DRIVING
FORCE, NOT AN OBSTACLE'

Bill Phillips

LITTLE BOOK OF
STRESS MANAGEMENT

What is Stress?	**3**
Awareness is the Key to Managing Stress	**5**
How do I know if I'm 'stressed out'?	
Recognising the Possible Signs of Stress	
Suggestions for Managers	**7**
What to look for	
What can be done to help?	
Suffering from Work or Home Related Stress?	**11**
Action Plan	
Ways to Manage Stress	**15**
Easy Stress Relievers	**19**
Feeling Blue? How Food can Help Lift Your Mood	**21**
Other Helpful Tips	
How Stressed are you in Your Daily Life?	**26**
Wheel of Life	**29**
Complementary Therapies	**31**

WHAT IS STRESS?

The Health and Safety Executive's formal definition of **work** related stress is:

"The adverse reaction people have to excessive pressures or other types of demand placed on them at work."

Stress is not an illness – it is a state. However, if stress becomes too excessive and prolonged, mental and physical illness may develop.

Work is generally good for people if it is well designed, but it can also be a great source of pressure. There is a difference between pressure and stress. Pressure can be positive; a motivating factor, and is often essential in a job. It can help us achieve our goals and perform better. Stress occurs when this pressure becomes excessive. Stress is a natural reaction to too much pressure.

In 2014-15 9.9 million working days were lost to stress, anxiety and depression in the UK alone.

www.hse.gov.uk/stress

The most common cause of stress is change. Not the actual change itself but how you approach it! If you believe you have no control over the situation it will increase your feelings of helplessness and anxiety.

Everybody experiences a certain amount of pressure. It is the body's natural reaction to tension and change. Some degree of pressure is good because it makes life challenging and less boring, however, stress is bad for you – both physically and mentally. Prolonged stress can lead to accidental injury or health problems such as; migraines, stroke, high blood pressure, heart disease, stomach ulcers, diabetes, back and skin problems (to name but a few).

For the sake of your health, safety and happiness, it is important to recognise and manage stress before it does you harm.

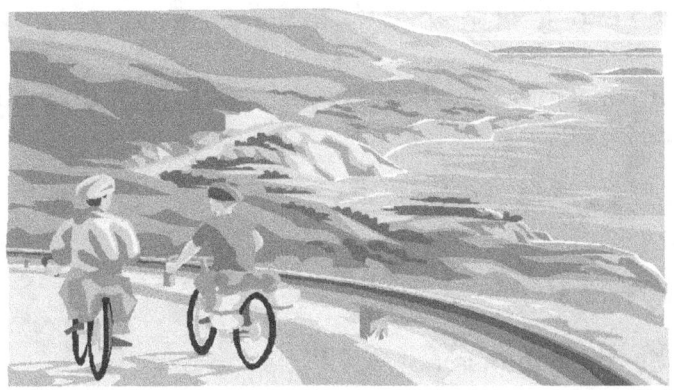

Take time out to do something you enjoy

AWARENESS IS THE KEY TO MANAGING STRESS

How do I know if I'm 'stressed out'?

- I hurt others with my words or actions.

- I reach out to things eg using alcohol, drugs or cigarettes, that seem to make the pain go away. This only works for a very short time.

- I just can't stop crying, everything hurts my feelings.

- I'm tired all the time and when I do get to sleep, I wake in the middle of the night with my head in a whirl.

- I'm a perfectionist, nothing is ever good enough; it's got to be perfect!

- I can't concentrate.

- I never seem to feel well these days.

- My motivation is not like it used to be.

- I have trouble breathing.

- I suffer from heart palpitations or panic attacks

Recognising the <u>Possible</u> Signs of Stress:

- Headaches
- Upset stomach
- Feeling uptight
- Anxiety
- Irritability
- Worrying too much
- Lack of energy
- Increased anger
- Poor concentration
- Skin, Nails and Hair condition deteriorate

- Changes in eating (eg more/less)
- Feeling powerless
- Sadness
- Difficulty sleeping
- Forgetfulness
- New/increased use of tobacco, alcohol or other drugs
- Hopelessness

If you find you suffer from several of these, you may be suffering from stress. Check out the Stress Test on pages 26 - 28.

Stress may be something felt by one person or a whole team/family. It has detrimental effects on both the individual and those around them.

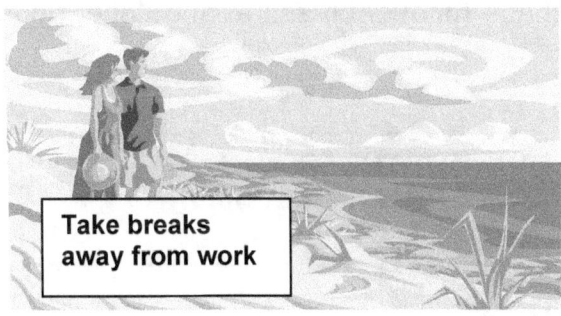

Take breaks
away from work

SUGGESTIONS FOR MANAGERS

What to look for:

- There is tension and conflict between certain colleagues.

- Sickness absence increases, often just odd days here and there for minor illnesses.

- Productivity and work performance drop. Motivation is poor.

- Time-keeping alters; the individual may take to working more hours, coming in late, etc.

- The person seems distracted.

- The person never has time to stop for a coffee, lunch etc as they feel they have too much to do.

What can be done to help?

- Consider how jobs and duties are organised in order to help manage undue pressure and long hours working.

> YOU ARE NOT THE PROGRAMME
> YOU ARE THE PROGRAMMER!
> ANON

"As a manager of a team of 8 I found that once we set clearly defined roles, where expectations placed on individuals were clear and non-conflicting; stress levels were dramatically reduced."

Robert

- Boring, repetitive work, too much or too little work, can lead to stress. Changing the way jobs are done helps. This can include moving people between jobs, giving staff more responsibility, increasing the scope of the job, increasing the variety of tasks, giving a group of workers greater responsibility for the effective performance of that group.

- Existing roles can often be split in new ways in order to accommodate staff at different grades and levels of seniority.

- If possible, provide some scope for varying working conditions and flexibility; and for people to influence the way their job is done. This will increase their sense of ownership and interest.

"I work in a team of 6. We find it really helpful that our new manager gives us notice of urgent and important jobs. This allows us to prioritise tasks. We have also identified and cut out unnecessary processes and streamlined our systems."

Emma

- It is important to remember that you need to value the quality as well as the quantity of work delivered.

- Many people will stay in the office or work at home if needs be. Sometimes managers, without realising it, take advantage of their staff's commitment.

- Ensure you acknowledge all staff commitment and not just those who are there during your working pattern. Acknowledging a job well done will help to improve staff morale.

"Ensure staff have the skills, training and resources they need to carry out their duties confidently and effectively. When I started my new job it was great to have a comprehensive induction plan from the start. It enabled me to quickly get to grips with my new role."

Mags

- Consider the needs and abilities of new recruits. There is a lead-in time before a person becomes fully effective. Concern about letting people down/not being effective, is very stressful. Remember to get a balance between the work undertaken and the knowledge of new recruits.

- Consider offering vouchers for complementary therapies or bringing in on-site massage etc to help staff de-stress at work

- If your new recruit is working late you may want to ensure that they are not feeling too much pressure and that they have the knowledge to undertake the job.

"The culture of 'blaming people when things go wrong' never works. By being honest with myself and my team, I think I'm setting a good example. We are now very open when things go wrong and we sort out any problems and issues together."

Justine

- Consider the expertise of individuals. It is not fair to expect people to do work for which they have neither the right expertise, nor the right training and then not support them. Neither is it fair to review their performance at the end of a period in a new post and judge them by the standards applied to long standing employees.

Ultimately show you take stress seriously and be understanding towards people who admit to being under too much pressure.

SHOOT FOR THE MOON. EVEN IF YOU MISS YOU'LL LAND AMONG THE STARS'
LES BROWN

Suffering from Work or Home Related Stress?

If you feel you cannot cope speak to someone in your support system such as your partner, a friend, your manager or your doctor.

Action Plan

A good way to help with managing pressure and achieving a healthier Life-Work Balance is to create an Action Plan. If work-related this could be included as part of an Appraisal process for yourself and for any staff you manage. Recognise that stress can be caused by placing expectations on both yourself and others that are too high to realistically meet.

Assess the situation and yourself - learn to recognise your own warning signs, these may include anxiety, withdrawal, mood swings or tearfulness. When you identify what your warning signs are, start employing some of the techniques identified in your plan.

> A DAY OF WORRY IS MORE EXHAUSTING
> THAN A WEEK OF WORK
>
> ANON

Your Action Plan may include:-

- A list of all the causes of stress that you recognise affect you. Often it is a number of factors combined rather than just one issue. Ask if you are contributing to your own stress levels. Look at each stressor and assess how you would deal with it

- Setting small steps to achieve quick-win solutions and giving yourself rewards/treats for achievements. These may include:

  o At work - take time to relax even though this is often the last thing on your priority list ie take a coffee break away from the desk or a short walk at lunch-time.

  o At home take time to read, take a bath, or do something else you find relaxing as a closure to your working day.

- Be realistic about your worries, include them in your plan. Many people waste a lot of time and create a lot of stress by worrying about things they have no control over. This creates the 'what if' cycle. This can often happen when there are not enough challenges in your life. Write down your worries - this may allow you to take more control of the situation.

Also remember:

- Try to ease body tension by having a good stretch and checking your posture from time to time.

- Don't balance your phone on your shoulder – invest in a headset.

- Ensure your work-area is well designed by conducting a risk assessment. Ergonomic work chairs are an asset if you can afford one.

- Take regular breaks especially if you are using a computer.

- If you feel you have to work at weekends, make it part of your Action Plan to work at the beginning of the weekend so that you have time for a definite break away from work. If you can, take some time out during the week to compensate.

*"Use your time wisely by establishing priorities. Make daily lists of what **must** be done, what **should** be done and what you **would like** to be done if there is time. Keep your list of goals achievable and divide big tasks into smaller ones. This really helped me focus on what I needed to achieve in that day and what could wait."*

Dominique

- It is ok to say "No"! If you are in a position to delegate, give other people a chance to accept the challenge from time to time.

"I found it really hard to say 'No' even when I knew it would be stressful for me. Once I actually started though it became easier and I was much less stressed as a result."
Vicki

- Ensure you take annual leave and enjoy it! Do not feel guilty about taking the time off. **This is especially important if you are self-employed.** We are all more effective if we allow ourselves to re-charge from time to time.

- Accept that you can't control everything; be flexible with yourself and others.

- Get yourself and your work-space organised. Cluttered work areas make for unnecessary stresses!

---

3 TIPS FOR SUCCESS:

- CELEBRATE YOUR ACHIEVEMENTS

- SHRUG OFF YOUR SETBACKS

- DEVELOP A SUPPORT NETWORK

Ways to Manage Stress

"I tried to think positively. It wasn't easy so I surrounded myself with others who were positive and supportive. I also put up positive sayings and calming pictures. It took time but it really did help."

Richard

- Be flexible. Know what you can change and what you can't. Go with the flow and be open to changes.

- Go ahead and make mistakes. No-one is perfect. The only way we really learn is from our mistakes. Accept them as the natural process of growing in wisdom. Use mistakes to learn – 'there is no failure only feedback'.

- Breathe slowly, deeply, and well. Some slow, deep breathing from your diaphragm really helps release stresses (see Easy Stress Relievers: Deep Breathing).

- Don't demand too much of yourself – asking for help is not a sign of weakness.

- 'If you feel anger and frustration then go and beat up a pillow – give vent to all that pent-up feeling too. Let it all out.

"Talk to others. Sharing life's difficulties and problems with a co-worker, friend, partner, or therapist, allows you to shed some of the weight of your burdens and to get a better perspective on things."

Trude

- Face your difficulties. Problems have a tendency to mount quickly until there can seem to be so many it is overwhelming. Your day will seem appreciably lighter after even one dreaded task is tackled so aim to start each day with at least one of these.

"I decided to change my eating habits. I started to eat more healthily, cutting down on refined sugar, which gives a quick hit of energy but leaves you feeling more tired than before. A healthy diet has increased my sense of well-being and I get far less minor illnesses now. I went on to cut out caffeine and to stop smoking as they were putting more stress on my nervous system."

Alan

Get More of These: **Try to Avoid These:**

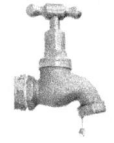
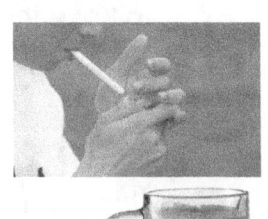
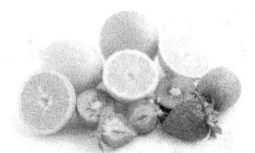
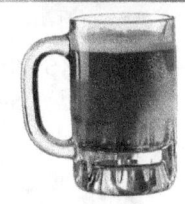
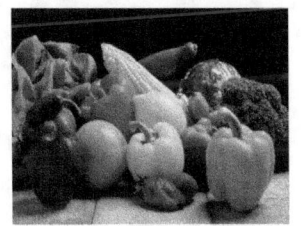
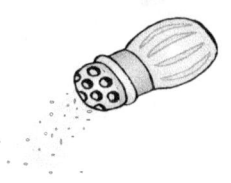

- Try to get plenty of sleep each night. If you can't sleep, don't lie there worrying. Get up and make yourself a hot non-caffeinated drink; do something repetitive and boring such as some ironing; or listen to a relaxation or hypnotherapy CD. Don't do something which stimulates you as this won't help you get back to sleep!

"I now try to make time for some exercise each day. It doesn't need to be strenuous, a gentle 10-15 minute walk at lunch time is enough to boost my energy levels and improve my mood. Exercise brings out the body's endorphins (those natural pain-killers and pleasure-producing chemicals produced inside every one of us)."

Suzanne

- If you feel like crying then let yourself cry. Allow yourself to have this emotional release.

"Make time to relax - listen to music, meditate, read, have a soothing bath, or do something else you enjoy. It really works for me when I give myself permission to do something just for ME."

Nadia

- Laugh and have fun. Play...with a partner, a friend, a child, a pet. Having fun is the natural way of lowering the body's stress hormones.

- Allow yourself to mourn. Changes, even good changes, can bring a sense of loss for how things used to be. You have the right to grieve this loss. In fact, everyone needs that time...to adjust, to reminisce, to care, to process.

"I found that as a care-giver, building a network of family members, friends, and neighbours who I can turn to in an emergency, or even just to give me a couple of hours break was invaluable. This network has become my safety valve."
Janet

- If you are a student, discuss your situation with your counsellor or tutor and identify ways you can continue to successfully work on your studies without burning out.

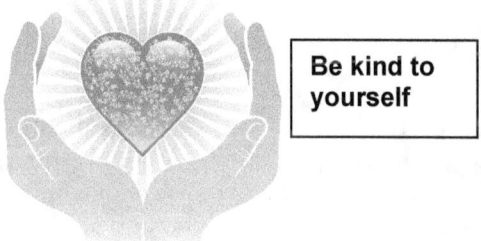

Be kind to yourself

Easy Stress Relievers

Deep Breathing

While in a comfortable position, take a long deep breath to the count of 3-6. Expand your stomach as far as you can. Hold for the count of 3. As you exhale to the count of 6, compress your stomach muscles and empty your lungs, imagine breathing in relaxation and breathing out all stress and tension. With each breath, think 'relax'. Do this several times, until you feel calmer.

Hum

Go on try it! Humming a tune causes relaxing vibrations in your throat.

Balloon Technique

Close your eyes and sit quietly. Imagine yourself standing in a hot-air balloon that is still on the ground. In the basket with you are bags of sand that represent your worries. As you toss each bag out of the basket onto the ground, the balloon begins to lift. When all the bags are gone, you are floating freely with no worries. Return when you are ready. Notice the change in your attitude.

Make a list

Writing down all your worries gets them out of your head. Once they are out, rip the list into as many pieces as you can and DUMP them in the bin or burn them.

Laugh

Watch or read something which makes you laugh. The harder you laugh, the less stressed you will feel. Try to do this at least once a day no matter how little you might feel like it before you start!

> TENSION IS WHO YOU THINK YOU SHOULD BE.
> RELAXATION IS WHO YOU ARE
> CHINESE PROVERB

FEELING BLUE?

How food can help lift your mood

Before we start

These pages are aimed at helping you get past those periodic 'blue' days we all experience from time to time, including SAD (Seasonal Affective Disorder). This is NOT a substitute for any prescription drugs you may be taking. If you are taking prescription drugs DO NOT come off them without first checking with your medical professional.

First the science

Research has shown that foods which contain the amino-acid tryptophan can help you to feel brighter, generally lift your mood and help you to sleep better. This is because tryptophan is broken down by your body into:-

A) Niacin which is anxiety reducing and sleep inducing,

and

B) Serotonin, which we all know is what gives us that feel good factor. It also controls sleep patterns, body temperature and sex drive.

Drugs such as Prozac work by artificially keeping the body's own serotonin levels high. You can achieve the same thing naturally – via your diet. You will need around 1000-2000 mg of tryptophan per day. Bearing in mind that tryptophan is one of the 10 essential amino acids you need to stay alive anyway you are well on the way to achieving your daily target without even being aware you are doing so.

The best source of serotonin is sunlight, so getting out whenever the sun is out is very beneficial; even in the winter. However, increased production in the brain is also triggered by St John's Wort. This is available on the high street and is frequently used by herbalists to treat mild to moderate depression. In Germany, it is prescribed three times more than Prozac!

To make serotonin, the body also needs a good supply of vitamin B6, which is found in carrots, fish, lentils, peas, potato, spinach and sunflower seeds - it is a good idea to increase your dietary intake of all these during the winter if you are prone to being SAD.

PEOPLE WHO DO NOT FIND TIME FOR
RECREATION ARE OBLIGED SOONER OR
LATER TO FIND TIME FOR ILLNESS
JOHN WANAMAKER

To get the tryptophan to that part of your body which will benefit most – your brain – eat plenty of carbohydrates with your tryptophan-loaded foods. Carbohydrates (potatoes, pasta, rice, bread etc) are required in order to cross the blood-brain barrier!

Vitamin C enables the body to convert the tryptophan into serotonin. Foods which contain high doses of vitamin C are blackcurrants, kiwi fruit, citrus fruits, onions, potatoes, sweet potatoes, cauliflower, tomatoes and green leafy vegetables. If you are looking for a high dose of vitamin C then look for Acerola Cherry supplements, (The Acerola Cherry contains 80 times more vitamin C than an orange weight for weight).

Which foods contain tryptophan?

Beans, cheese, nuts and seeds, poultry, grains, eggs and brewer's yeast all contain good proportions of tryptophan per portion. The measure of the portions listed below is per 100 grams (3.5 oz). This is not a lot so you might easily double or treble the figures listed below in just one meal.

NB. Just because a variety of something listed on the next page is not mentioned it does not mean it does not contain tryptophan. Baked potatoes (if you also eat the skins) contain high doses but we do not have access to the actual figures per 100g.

Beans	mg/100g	Cheese	
Lentils	215	Cheddar	340
Dried Peas	250	**Parmesan**	**490**
Baked	210	Swiss-type	375
Kidney	215		
Soya	**525**	Other cheeses tend to be lower in	
Nuts and seeds		Tryptophan but are still good	
Brazil Nuts	185	**Poultry**	250
Cashews	**470**		
Hazelnuts	210	**Eggs**	210
Peanuts	340		
Pumpkin seeds	**560**	**Brewers Yeast**	**700**
Sesame seeds	330	**Meats**	
Tahini	**575**		
Sunflower seeds	340	Meat is generally regarded as a good source of tryptophan, however most meats range from 160-260, with offal reaching up to 330.	
Other nuts	130 +		
Grains			
Wheatgerm	265		

Other Helpful Tips:

In the Middle East, Basil is made into a tea that is taken to relieve mild depression. It also has a long history in Ayurvedic medicine as a good herb for the treatment of nervous disorders and anxiety. In aromatherapy, Basil essential oil can even have a mildly sedative effect.

The Bedouin use Frankincense as an anti-depressant; consider burning the resin or the essential oil to benefit from these properties.

Exercise is an excellent antidote to the blues since working the body   releases endorphins. As we are aware, these are the body's own feel-good chemicals that create a natural feeling of well-being. The British Heart Foundation recommends 5 x 30 minute sessions per week. It does not have to be strenuous, walking is great, particularly if you raise your pace a little (make sure you can still keep up a conversation or the pace is too fast!)

> 'PEOPLE ARE LIKE STAINED-GLASS WINDOWS.
> THEY SPARKLE AND SHINE WHEN THE SUN IS OUT,
> BUT WHEN THE DARKNESS SETS IN, THEIR TRUE
> BEAUTY IS REVEALED ONLY IF THERE IS A LIGHT
> FROM WITHIN."
> ELIZABETH KUBLER ROSS

How Stressed are you in your Daily Life?

Here are some questions which will reflect how stressed you are in daily life – tick each column which most clearly reflects how true this is for you most of the time, and then add up your scores.

In the last few months how often have you:

	Often	Some-times	Seldom	Never
Lost your appetite?				
Found you are constantly nibbling at sugary snack foods?				
Felt sick after eating?				
Bitten your nails?				
Been restless and fidgety?				
Found yourself getting angry or upset for little or no reason?				
Felt you HAVE to work extra hard or late more often?				
Been worked up by heavy traffic or other travellers?				
Tried harder to win in sports?				
Tried harder to win in arguments?				
Struggled for perfection?				

	Often	Some-times	Seldom	Never
Felt that you don't spend enough time with your family?				
Found it difficult to sleep at night?				
Used alcohol when under pressure?				
Used cigarettes or drugs to help when you are under pressure?				
Felt trapped by your lifestyle?				
Found you are too busy to do things you enjoy doing?				
Found it hard to make decisions?				
Worried about your future?				
Found it hard to concentrate?				
Suffered from headaches?				
Found yourself grumbling or moaning almost constantly?				
Found it difficult to laugh or smile or think positively about your life?				

Now add up the number of ticks in each column. **TOTAL TICKS**				
Then multiply each column by	x3	x2	x1	x0
Add the four columns together:	**GRAND TOTAL =**			

Now check your results!

<u>Quiz Scores</u>

If you have **more than 45** then your stress level is high! You may be a workaholic and you may be suffering from the physical effects of stress. You definitely need to manage your stress levels **NOW.** Use the useful tips in this book to help you.

If you have **between 35 and 44** then your stress level is still too high. You need to manage your stress levels before they get any higher!

If you have **between 25 and 34** then your stress level is moderate but it is worth learning how to relax more so that you build your energy reserves for when you need them.

A score of **below 25** indicates that you have got the balance about right! You show few signs of stress but keep checking it stays that way.

Adapted from 'Your guide to Understanding Stress' by Stress Check

The Wheel of Life

Directions: The eight segments represent balance. Firstly you can rename any of the segments to make the wheel more appropriate to you. Then consider the centre of the wheel as 0 and the outer rim as 10 and rank your satisfaction in each area of your life by drawing a line and creating your personal wheel (see the second diagram below). Once completed - how bumpy would this ride be if it were a real wheel?

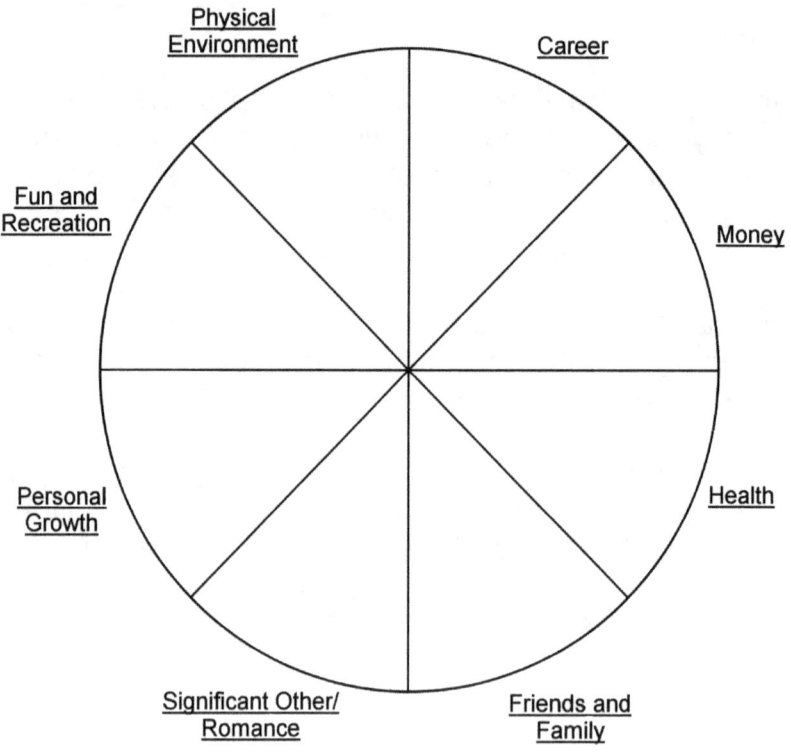

Now you know which segments you need to work on to address any imbalances you may have in your life!

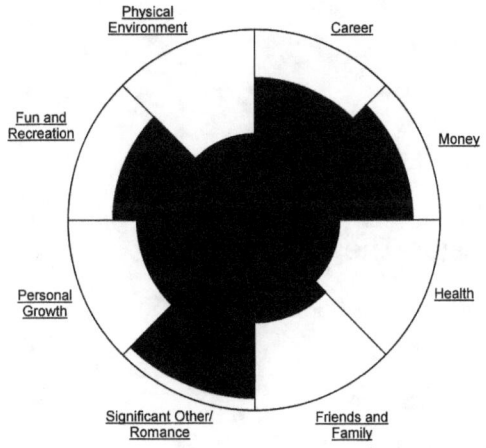

An example of an out-of-balance wheel of life.

Complementary Therapies and Activities You May Find Beneficial:

- Acupuncture/Acupressure
- Alexander Technique
- Aromatherapy
- Aura-Soma
- Bach's Flower Remedies
- Bowen Technique
- Cranio-Sacral Therapy
- Clinical Hypnotherapy
- Energy Healing: Ascension Therapy, Reiki etc
- Hopi Ear Candling
- Herbal Medicine
- Homeopathy
- Massage
- Meditation classes and CDs
- Pilates
- Reflexology
- Shiatsu
- Yoga

Love Your Life also have an MP3 available to help you manage stress more effectively. It can be purchased from www.love-yourlife.co.uk

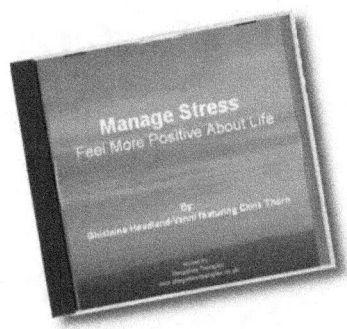

You can find out more about Love Your Life at:

Facebook: https://www.facebook.com/LoveYrLife
Twitter: https://twitter.com/luvyourlife2
Instagram: https://www.instagram.com/luvyourlife
Pinterest: https://uk.pinterest.com/luvyourlife2/
LinkedIn: https://www.linkedin.com/in/loveyourlife
Blogger: http://luvyourlife2.blogspot.co.uk